THROUGH THE EYES OF A SURVIVOR -
TRAUMATIC BRAIN INJURY

THROUGH THE EYES OF A SURVIVOR -
TRAUMATIC BRAIN INJURY

Brian Maram

Copyright

THROUGH THE EYES OF A SURVIVOR –
TRAUMATIC BRAIN INJURY

Copyright © 2022 Brian Maram

First edition 2022

The author has made every effort to trace and
acknowledge sources/resources/individuals. In the
event that any images/information have been
incorrectly attributed or credited, the Author will be
pleased to rectify these omissions at the earliest
opportunity

Self-Published by: Brian Maram

Website: www.neuvare.com

Cover designed by: Brian Maram

E-mail: info@neuvare.com

Dedication

"To my loving children
Thank you for your
support and patience, I
would never have achieved
my dream without your
encouragement."

Disclaimer

This book is a work of non-fiction and is intended to provide accurate information in regards to the subject matter covered. The content is based on factual information provided to and by the author, and any similarities to other individuals, real, fictional, dead or alive are purely coincidental.

This book is not intended to be used, nor should it be used, to diagnose or treat any medical condition. For diagnosis or treatment of any medical problem, consult your own physician. The editor, publisher and author are not responsible for any specific health or allergy needs that may require medical supervision and are not liable for any damages or negative consequences from any treatment, action, application or preparation, to any person reading or following the information in this book. Neither is this book intended as a substitute for the medical advice of physicians. The reader should regularly consult a physician in matters relating to his/her/their health and particularly with respect to any symptoms that may require diagnosis or medical attention.

This book is designed based on the author's personal experience and is meant to provide information and motivation to its readers. It is sold with the understanding that the publisher and author are not engaged to render any type of medical, psychological, legal, or any other kind of professional advice. The content is the sole

Acknowledgements

"I would like to thank my children and therapists without whose dedicated help and support this book would never have been completed."

Table of Contents

Preface

If you are reading this book, you have either survived a life-changing Traumatic Brain Injury or you know someone who has.

Inevitably, the family will be overjoyed that their loved one survived such a horrendous ordeal. Little do they realise how unprepared they are for the complex flood of emotions the survivor is about to unleash on them.

Surviving a TBI is the easy part, but the life-changing ordeal that is about to follow will ultimately put the entire family through one of hell's more definitive tests. As you embark on this new unpredictable journey, the life you once knew is about to end, and the one that lies ahead of you is a life you could never have imagined. With no instruction manuals to guide you through this treacherous journey, you will find yourself having to wing it as you go.

The author, a TBI survivor himself, survived a head-on collision when a drunk driver failed to stop at an intersection. From that dreadful moment, the lives of his close-knit family were changed forever. No one was prepared for the mystifying flood of emotions that were about to be set into motion.

Lucky to be alive, he was rushed to hospital. After an emergency operation, he was placed into an induced coma in ICU. The impact from the collision had caused the author to suffer a Traumatic Brain Injury.

The years that followed were pure hell for his family, and after numerous therapy sessions and operations, he made a full recover

CHAPTER ONE

Brain Anatomy

Brain Structure

The brain is a complex organ and is divided into three principal areas, consisting of the Cerebrum, Cerebellum and Brainstem.

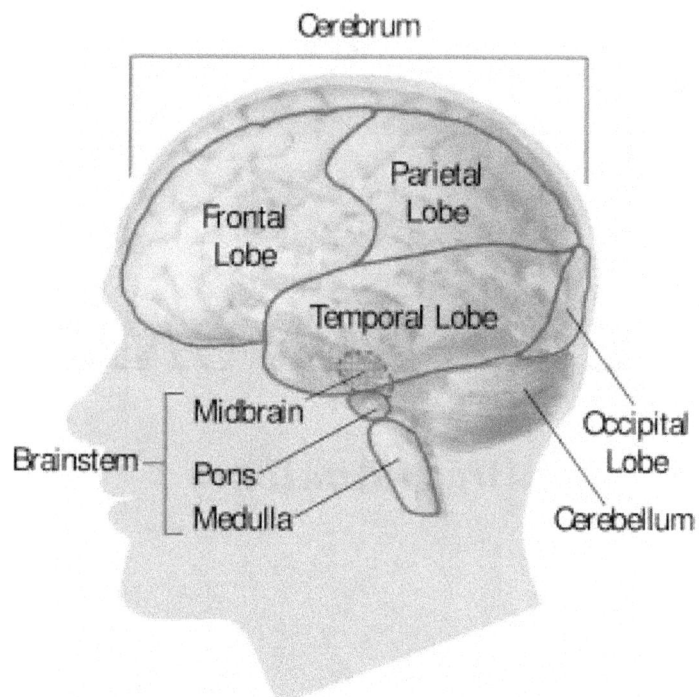

The largest part of the human brain is the Cerebrum which is divided into two hemispheres and is associated with higher brain function. Each hemisphere is made up of four lobes consisting of the Frontal, Temporal, Parietal and Occipital Lobes.

These four lobes are then further subdivided into

substructures that are associated with specific functions which have been detailed below under each description.

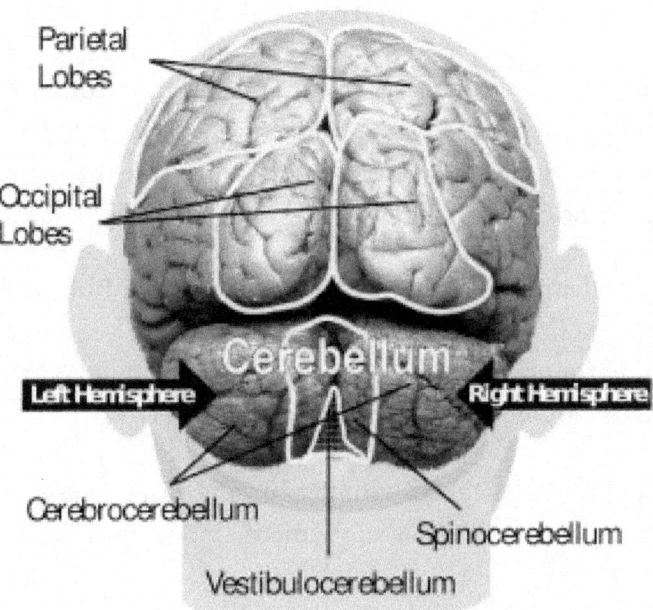

The Cerebellum is located at the brain's posterior and is positioned under the cerebrum hemispheres.

The brainstem is situated deep inside the brain and is a continuance of the spinal cord. The Pons, Medulla Oblongata and Midbrain make up the brainstem.

The **left hemisphere** of the brain controls the right side of the body and is responsible for **speech, comprehension, arithmetic, and writing**.

The right hemisphere controls the left side of the body and is responsible for creativity, spatial ability, artistic, and musical skills.

Frontal Lobe

The Frontal Lobes can be found in the front of the brain and makes up the largest portion of the brain. Forming part of the cerebral cortex, it is the main site for higher cognitive functioning.

The substructures that make up the Frontal Lobe are the prefrontal cortex, orbitofrontal cortex, motor and premotor cortices, Broca's area, frontal eye fields, middle and inferior frontal gyru.

Functions associated with the Frontal Lobe play a major part in one's voluntary movement.

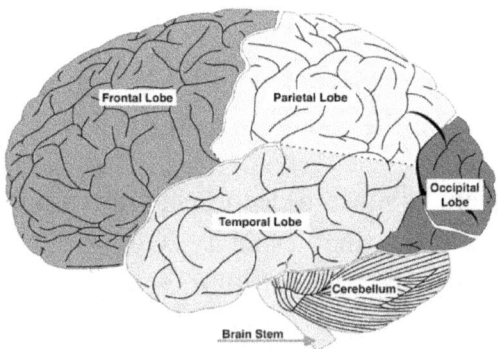

Activities such as walking are controlled by the Frontal Lobe as it houses the primary motor cortex.

Other functions include: executive procedures (decision-making skills, planning, problem-solving, judgement, inhibition and thinking), attention and thought, voluntary behaviour, cognition, intelligence, language processing and comprehension, plus many more.

Damage to the Frontal Lobe might cause paralysis, mood changes and nonconforming social and personality behaviours. Emotions that are felt by the survivor, may not necessarily be expressed in their face or voice. On the contrary, they may exhibit excessive displays of emotions.

Parietal Lobe

The substructures making up the Parietal Lobe are the somatosensory cortex, inferior and superior parietal lobules and the praecuneus.

Functions associated with the Parietal Lobe include perception and integration of somatosensory information (touch, pressure pain and temperature), visuospatial processing, spatial attention and mapping, as well as number representation.

Damage to the Parietal Lobe could cause the inability to locate and recognise objects, hemispatial neglect (a lack of attention to and awareness of one side of the field of vision), disorientation and lack of coordination.

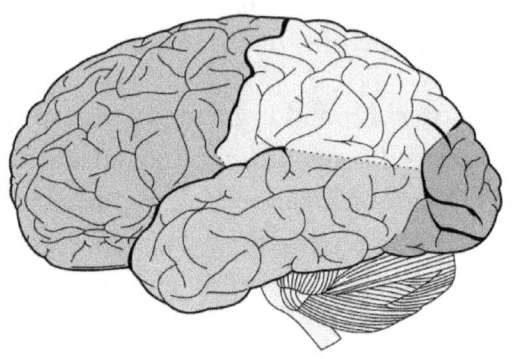

Temporal Lobe

The Temporal Lobe consists of several substructures. These include the amygdala, the primary auditory cortex, superior and middle temporal gyrus, Wernicke's area and the fusiform gyrus.

Functions associated with the Temporal Lobe include perception (hearing, vision, smell), face recognition, learning and memory, understanding of language and emotional reactions.

Damage to the Temporal Lobe may result in difficulties in understanding speech (Wernicke's Aphasia), recognition of faces and objects, the inability to attend to sensory input, persistent talking, memory loss (short and long term), an increase or decrease in sexual behaviour, aggression and difficulty recalling visual stimuli.

Dysfunction of the Temporal Lobe is closely aligned with the neuropathological disorder, Schizophrenia.

Occipital Lobe

The two Occipital Lobes are the smallest of the four paired lobes in the cerebral cortex. The primary visual area of the brain is located in the Occipital cortex. Because it's the primary visual centre, it contains most of the anatomical region of the visual cortex and its substructures consist of the cuneus and visual areas V1 – V5.

The Occipital Lobe is associated with vision and d*amage* to this area could result in hallucinations, blindness and the inability to see colour or motion.

Cerebellum

The Cerebellum is the region of the brain that coordinates and regulates motor behaviour, particularly automatic movements. It is located at the bottom of the brain and is tucked in under the cerebral hemispheres.

Functions associated with the Cerebellum include voluntary movement, motor learning, reflex, balance memory, posture, timing and sequence learning.

Damage to this area of the brain could result in the loss

of coordination, tremors, inability to walk, dizziness (vertigo) or slurred speech.

Brainstem

The Brainstem is situated in the posterior part of the brain and is a continuation of the spinal cord. It is made up of structures that lie deep within the brain and consists of the pons, medulla oblongata and midbrain.

It plays a vital role in maintaining and controlling automated functions such as breathing, blood pressure and heart rate. It further regulates the central nervous system and is crucial in maintaining consciousness.

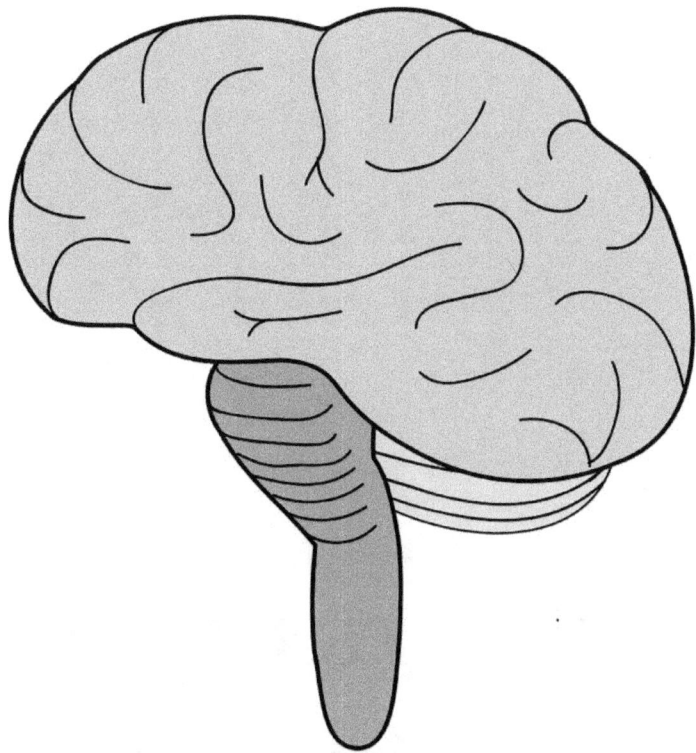

The Brainstem is *associated with* the body's automated functions (blood pressure, breathing, heartbeat, digestion, perspiration and temperature), as well as alertness, sleep, balance and the startle response.

Damage to this area could cause organ failure, resulting in death, sleep disorders (such as insomnia or sleep apnoea), difficulties with balance and moving.

CHAPTER TWO

Hospitalisation

MRI

Magnetic resonance imaging (MRI) is a medical imaging technique used in radiology to form pictures of the body's anatomy and physiological processes.

An MRI can detect various brain conditions, *especially following head trauma.* Conditions such as bleeding, swelling, inflammation or problems with the blood vessels. An MRI can also detect cysts, tumours, developmental and structural abnormalities and infections in patients.

The MRI scanner is a large cylindrical tube that contains powerful magnets, and patients are passed through the inside of the tube during the scan.

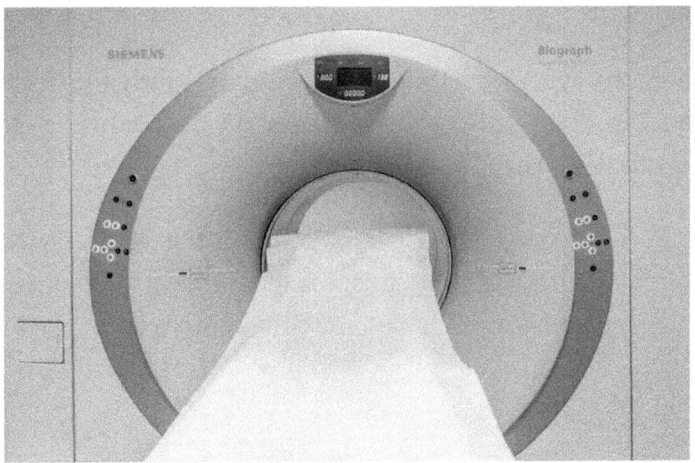

They help doctors identify what is causing a patient's health issue and to diagnose them accurately, allowing them to prescribe a treatment plan. Depending on a patient's symptoms, an MRI can be used to scan a specific portion of their body for diagnosing, for example, only the brain in the case of a TBI patient. An MRI can also help doctors to identify structural lesions.

Computerised Tomography (CT)

A **computerised tomography (CT)** scan combines a series of X-ray images taken from various angles and uses computer processing to create cross-sectional images (slices) of bones, blood vessels and soft tissues inside a patient's body. They reveal internal injuries and bleeding, such as those caused by Traumatic Brain Injury. The images from a CT scan are more detailed than that of standard X-rays and are painless, fast and easy.

X-rays, MRIs, and CT scans can detect fractures, haemorrhages, swelling, and certain kinds of tissue damage, but unfortunately, **they do not always see traumatic brain injuries**.

A non-contrast head CT is displayed in head trauma patients with loss of consciousness or post-traumatic amnesia in the presence of specific symptoms.

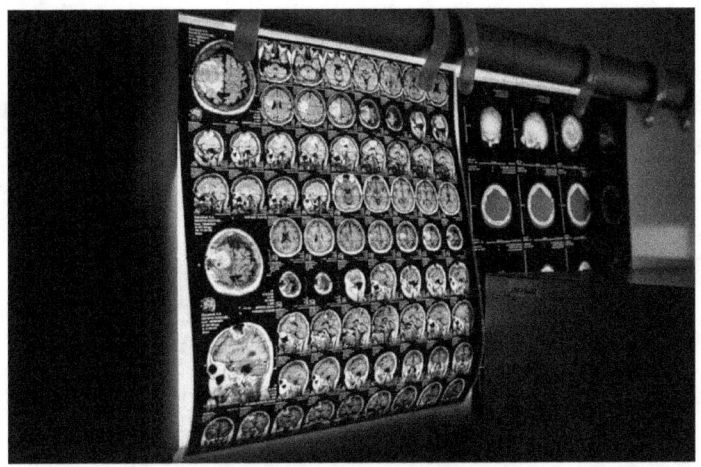

The radiation exposure is small with one head scan. But repeated exposure to scans over a long period can increase the patient's cancer risk. Today's CT scan technology is more advanced than those of the past and faster than what it used to be. Therefore, the radiation exposure is even **less than it once** was.

That First Hospital Visit

Visiting a loved one in the hospital for the first time can be a traumatic experience. It can be overwhelming to see a loved one helplessly lying in bed, entangled in a web of pipes and cables and hanging onto life.

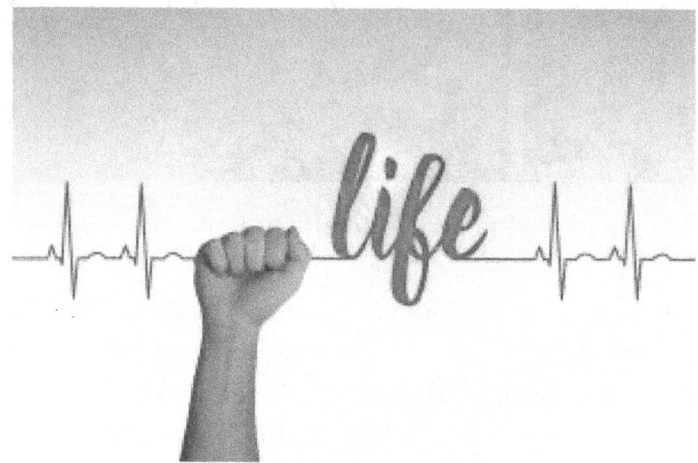

The patient may be in a coma and unresponsive due to the head trauma. The uncertainty of what the future holds can be daunting as everything will be up uncertain until such time that they awake. It is only then can the true extent of the damage be accessed.

Once exposed to TBI, the lives of the survivor, their family and friends are thrown into turmoil. The devastation unleashed onto them is overwhelming and surprisingly fast. Life changes instantaneously, and the injury can come at a tremendous cost, both financially and health-wise, impacting your independence and relationships.

Not many people realise the extended impact a brain injury can have on the family; overnight, a partner becomes a caregiver or a breadwinner becomes unemployable. The life you once knew abruptly comes to a screeching halt. In a flash of light, lives are changed forever and forever is a long time to try and envisage.

No books or publications could ever truly prepare a family for the life they are about to find themselves in.

Stripped of their independence, the aftermath of a brain injury is devastating and approached with fear and anticipation. Apprehension and uncertainty now taint the future of those close to the survivor. With no idea what lies ahead of them, families fear the worst, as they anxiously step into uncharted waters.

Those close to the patient will be caught off guard by the tsunami of emotions that are about to come flooding in and will be unfamiliar with what to look out for. Not knowing how to handle the situation on their own, they will desperately need assistance from a **neuro-psychologist.** A neuropsychologist has a better understanding of the impact a head injury can have on a patient.

Stabilisation

The hospital's priority following a brain injury is to stabilise the patient. Once the hospitalised survivor is medically stable, the hospital can then move them to inpatient rehabilitation.

Inpatient rehabilitation is also referred to as acute rehabilitation.

Patients who cannot meet the requirements of inpatient rehabilitation may be discharged to a skilled nursing facility.

CHAPTER THREE

Nursing Facility

Skilled Nursing Facility

The difference between a nursing home and a skilled nursing facility is whether they offer medical care or not.

People with acute conditions requiring **medical care**, such as stroke or TBI survivors, would be sent to a skilled nursing facility.

Skilled nursing facilities (SNF) are establishments for the elderly or disabled who require medical care and cannot look after themselves. Nursing facilities may also be referred to as nursing homes, skilled nursing facilities, long-term care facilities, old age homes, assisted living facilities, care homes, rest homes, convalescent homes or convalescent care. The titles differ slightly to indicate the levels of care offered and whether the institution is public or private.

They also indicate whether they provide mainly assisted living, only nursing care or nursing care with emergency medical care.

Skilled Nursing facilities are the solution for patients who do not need to be in a hospital but cannot be cared for at home.

Nurses are responsible for the caring of a patients' medical needs at nursing facilities. Depending on their rank and seniority, the responsibilities of the nurse may extend to being in charge of other employees. Skilled nursing facilities have nursing aides and experienced nurses on hand 24/7.

Nursing Home

People who require assistance with everyday living tasks and **non-medical care** would go to a nursing home.

Nursing facilities also go by many different names depending on their levels of care. They may be referred to as nursing homes, long-term care facilities, old age homes, assisted living facilities, care homes, rest homes, convalescent homes or convalescent care. The titles will differ slightly to indicate the levels of care on offer and whether the institution is public or private.

The name is indicative of whether they provide mainly assisted living with nursing care or nursing care with emergency medical care.

Nurses are also responsible for caring for a resident's medical needs at nursing homes.

CHAPTER FOUR

Understanding TBI

Neurological Insults

Head injuries are serious, fear-provoking medical emergencies, which have a daunting effect on the entire family. They are unpredictable life-changing, and most survivors and their loved ones will have no idea where to turn or what is involved in the recovery process.

Head traumas are not something you plan for in your life; no individual of sound mind would place head trauma and disability on their bucket list. It's something that happens when life takes control, unexpectedly and usually in the blink of an eye.

When non-fatal, the survivors are often left with debilitating disabilities that could have devastating consequences that could impoverish an entire family.

To cope with the repercussions of the injury, families and survivors (if capable) need to be well-informed. Despite what has happened, it's imperative to remember that no two head injuries are alike.

If you know someone who has survived a Traumatic Brain Injury, then your claim to fame is that you know someone who has survived a Traumatic Brain Injury. Knowing what to anticipate during a survivor's recovery is a mystery to everyone.

The services of a professional will address any fears or concerns stemming from these uncertain times. Recovering from a head trauma requires the dedicated assistance of numerous doctors and therapists, each one experienced in their field.

Traumatic Brain Injury (TBI)

A TBI is a traumatically induced structural injury and/or physiological disruption of brain function as a result of an external force that is characterised by the onset or the worsening of at least one of the following clinical signs directly following an of the below events:

- Any loss of or decrease in consciousness
- Any loss of memory for events immediately before or after the injury
- Any change in mental state at the time of the injury (i.e. confusion, disorientation, slowed thinking, etc.)
- Any neurological deficits (weakness, loss of balance, change in vision, praxis, paresis/plegia, sensory loss, aphasia, etc.) that may or may not be temporary
- Intracranial lesion
- External forces such as:
  - the head being struck by an object
  - the head striking an object
  - the brain undergoing an acceleration/ deceleration movement without direct external trauma to the head
  - a foreign object penetrating the skull/ brain
  - The shock wave generated by a blast or explosion

- o Injuries caused during sports activities
- o Injuries caused by falls (common in the elderly and toddlers)

No matter the cause, that person has experienced a traumatic brain injury. The consequences of such an injury could range from mild to devastatingly severe.

Contact sports injuries and car accidents account for a large number of Traumatic brain injuries.

Improved medical emergency care over the years has resulted in a decrease in the mortality rate amongst TBI patients; as a result, it has increased the morbidity rate. Increasing the number of people now living with neurological impairments.

This has had a significant impact on economies when considering the hospitalisation, rehabilitation, medication, and the loss of working hours. More importantly, the emotional burden is unknown; it is impossible to place a value on the emotional impact it would have on patients and those close to the survivor.

Acquired Brain Injury (ABI)

An acquired brain injury is an injury to the brain that occurred after birth but is not related to a congenital defect or degenerative disease.

Causes of ABI include (but are not limited to) hypoxia, illness, infection, Cerebrovascular accident ((CVA) aka stroke), substance abuse, toxic exposure, and tumour.

ABI's can cause temporary or permanent impairment in cognitive, emotional, metabolic, motor, perceptual-motor and/or sensory brain function.

Surviving A Brain Injury

Whether it's acquired or traumatic, surviving a brain injury is the easy part when a survivor has the desire to live. However, the weeks, months and even years that follow are where the demanding challenges lie. After rigorous in-patient rehabilitation, survivors are discharged and released back into an unforgiving society. A society that does not understand what they have had to endure.

Leaving the safe confines of the rehabilitation centre, survivors and their families are expected to fend for themselves. Oblivious to the chaos the injury is about to unleash on their lives. Unknowingly, they will take their loved ones home, oblivious to what lies ahead of them. The world they once knew has been shattered and is about to be turned upside down. What they once took for granted is about to become a distant memory. Trapped in a life they had not anticipated, families are left to their own and expected to unearth the complexity of their inconceivable future.

With their lives already in shambles, the family is about to encounter circumstances that they could never have anticipated or envisioned. With turmoil and confusion now at the core of their existence, they will desperately begin to seek direction.

Survivors are often lunged back into their infant years and will require continuous attention, disrupting the once serene home that they had grown accustomed to. The imminent sacrifices are abundant, and one of the toughest you will encounter is for a family member to resign from their job and take on the caregiver's responsibility. Doing so may not be a plausible option, especially with all those exorbitant, accumulating medical bills, but rather a necessity. Hiring a full-time caregiver may not be an option either, as they also cost money and only contribute to the already copious medical bills.

In addition to the substantial financial burdens, the family would be placing all their trust in a stranger by inviting them into their lives and home to take care of their already vulnerable loved one.

Neurological disorders are growing at an alarming rate and are not limited to stroke and TBI. They extend over a vast array of conditions, such as Multiple Sclerosis (MS), Autism, Cerebral Palsy (CP), Dementia, Alzheimer's Disease, and even incomplete spinal cord injuries, to mention just a few.

Different Types Of TBI

There are two different types of TBI. Both are serious and should be treated as so. The two are:

- **Closed brain injury**. These injuries occur when there is a non-penetrating injury to the brain. i.e. there is no break in the cranium/skull.
- **Penetrating brain injury**. On the other hand. Penetrating or open brain injuries occur when the cranium/skull is fractured. An example would be when a bullet pierces the brain.

Common Cause Of TBI

A common cause of TBI is from falls.

Be it from tripping, falling out of bed, off a ladder, down the stairs or in the bath.

The majority of these TBIs are amongst the elderly and young children. Both are susceptible to falls.

Traumatic brain injuries are not restricted to MVA's (motor vehicle accidents). Due to the many unfortunate and high profile injuries in sports over the past few years, the awareness of traumatic brain injury has increased worldwide.

TBIs include concussions, which result from a blow to the head or may be caused by effectively shaking the brain.

Can Brain Damage Be Reversed?

While **damage to the brain cannot be reversed**, functions affected by TBI can be recovered thanks to the brain's amazing natural ability to rewire itself through a process known as neuroplasticity.

Please see neuroplasticity under Living with a TBI survivor.

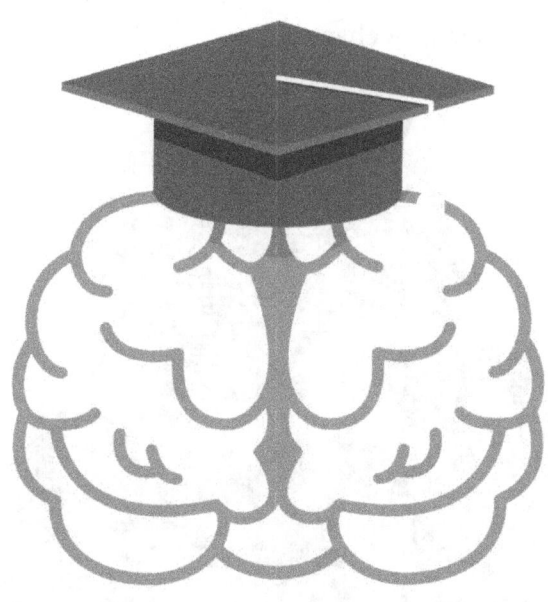

Are There Personality Changes In TBI Patients?

Head injuries cause damage to the brain, and patients can lose control over their emotions.

This condition has a name and so it is not uncommon. It is known as emotional liability, and it plays a part in how patients react to certain situations.

Emotional liability plays a significant role in how a patient's personality changes.

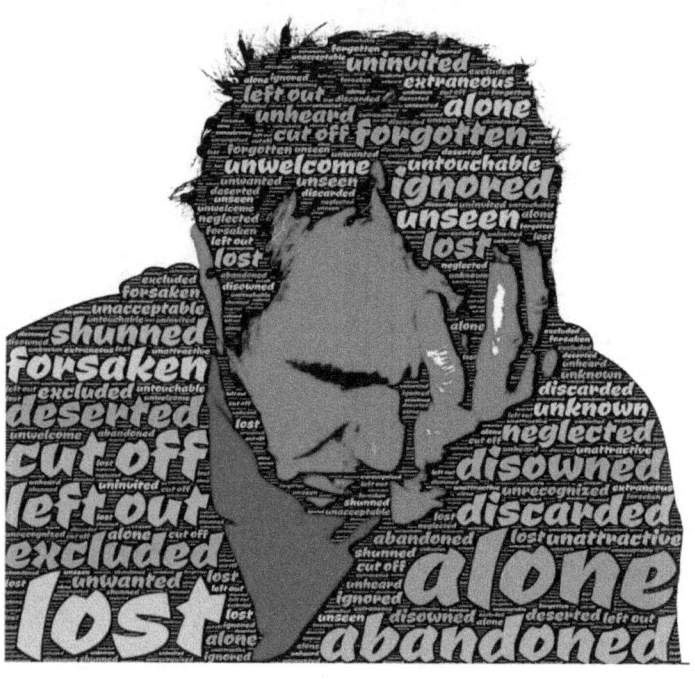

Do Patients Recover From TBI?

Depending on the severity of the TBI, patients can and do recover from mild TBI.

Usually, it takes between a week to three months, depending on the severity. The older the patient, the longer it may take, especially if they are over 40.

Patients can and do recover from Severe TBI, but it does take longer.

Patients can remain unconscious for days, weeks or even years. Some injuries are so severe that patients never recover from their disabilities.

Severe TBIs are responsible for thousands of deaths each year. Those who survive severe TBI usually lead a life with physical, cognitive, emotional and /or behavioural issues.

Each injury is unique and beyond comparison, and patients that do recover do so at different rates.

Can Severe TBI Shorten Your Life Span?

Surviving a moderate to severe TBI increases a patient's risk of dying earlier by about nine years. This is compared to people without TBI.

Those with TBI typically inherit various chronic health

conditions and are at higher risk and more susceptible to dying from seizures, drug poisoning, infections or pneumonia.

Can You Recover From Paralysis After A Traumatic Brain Injury?

Damage to the brain is permanent and cannot be reversed—through a process known as neuroplasticity, and with intensive therapy, patients experiencing hemiplegia or hemiparesis can regain some of the motion and movement back that they lost due to their injury.

Several rehabilitation techniques can combat post-injury paralysis.

See Neuroplasticity under Living with a TBI survivor.

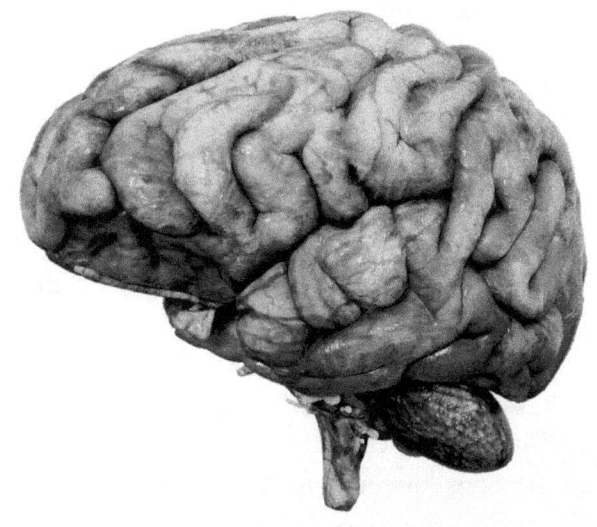

The New Normal

What is normal?

What might be considered normal to one person may not be perceived as normal to another.

Define normal?

Normal is ....

Surviving a Traumatic Brain Injury with complete or incomplete paralysis is devastating to the survivor and everybody close to them.

The world you all formerly knew has abruptly ended, and that "normal" life you once relished has taken on an entirely new meaning.

Surviving such a frightening ordeal will undoubtedly leave all of you feeling delighted that your loved one is alive.

Bear in mind that the survivor may no longer be able to contend with life's chores as effectively as they once did.

In its wake of destruction, the injury may have caused overwhelming, irreversible damage to the brain, with devastating consequences for the survivor, forcing them to take on life in a new type of 'normal' way.

How is anyone expected to know what to anticipate without an instruction manual to follow?

All brain injuries are unique, and no two injuries can be compared.

The best advice that I can give you is that you need to realise that what the survivor had before the trauma may have disappeared forever.

It is now time for you to re-evaluate their situation. Take stock of what has been exhausted and what remains. Once you know what's remaining, you have identified the foundation on which to start building.

Survivors now need to focus all their attention on what remains and progressively start rehabilitating themselves from here.

Emotional Liability

Nothing can prepare you for the complex surge of emotions the survivor is about to unleash on you.

Having survived such an ordeal, they might seem like a stranger to you. Initially, the overwhelming shock of what has happened will cause them to struggle with their emotions.

Survivors are prone to intense feelings and sudden mood swings, a condition referred to as emotional liability.

A survivor's emotional liability may be out of sync with their current environment, and it may bring on the Pseudobulbar Affect (PBA).

Pseudobulbar Affect (PBA)

The abundance of emotional liability that is building up could bring on the **Pseudobulbar Affect (PBA)**, a medical condition characterised by the sudden and uncontrollable occurrences of laughter or crying, without any apparent motivating stimulus.

PBA is usually inappropriate behaviour to the current situation. A survivor may find themselves laughing uncontrollably at an unhappy situation or crying uncontrollably at a joyful event.

CHAPTER FIVE

Living with a TBI survivor

Home Modifications

Modifications to the home will be necessary to accommodate the survivor's needs whilst ensuring their safety.

Depending on the severity of the TBI and if there is paralysis, they may need a wheelchair. If this is the case, modifications will need to be done to the home to accommodate the wheelchair.

One of the most hazardous rooms in the home is the bathroom. With its numerous sharp edges and slippery floors, grab rails will be necessary and should be fitted in strategic places, like inside the shower and adjacent to the toilet.

A hand shower and a non-slip shower chair will also be required for the survivor to bathe safely. Clearing an area adjacent to the toilet will be necessary to allow easy access for the wheelchair and unrestricted transferring if they are alone.

Furniture and loose rugs should be moved around or placed into storage, allowing for easy access of the survivor and their wheelchair. Once the survivor begins to walk, those lose rugs and mats will become hazardous obstacles if left in place.

If you have stairs in the home, a ramp may be necessary. But before installing any permanent features, ensure that you have done your homework and that the angles are correct. After all, everything to be installed is to ensure the survivor's safety at the end of the day.

The kitchen is filled with many sharp and dangerous utensils. If the crockery and utensils they need are out of reach, they should be relocated for easy access. Areas may also have to be cleared up here to allow for the safe passage of the wheelchair.

Buffer Zone

With so much uncertainty and concern, it is natural for friends and family to call or request media updates on how the survivor is doing.

A family member or close friend should step in at this point and act as a go-between. *They need to create a zone of tranquillity around the survivor.*

Stress And Recovery

This chapter in the survivor's life is challenging, and recovery is a painstakingly slow process.

Try to keep any additional stress to an ultimate minimum, as any extra pressure will further hamper the recovery process.

Informal Caregivers

A survivor might not be able to perform specific tasks that came to them naturally in the past.

Things will usually only begin to improve with a prolonged recovery process, and this will occur once the healing process has begun.

Your job as a Caregiver is to be there for them. Help them along this unpleasant journey by making them feel loved. Showing love and affection is vital to speeding up the recovery process.

As a Caregiver, it is your responsibility to let them know that you feel strongly about them and that taking unnecessary risks where their life and safety are concerned is not acceptable.

As a caregiver, it is important that you also look after your health and well-being.

Evidence has shown that most informal caregivers are ill-prepared for this role and provide care with little to no support—*more than one-third of them who continue to provide intense care land up jeopardising their health.*

Caregiving is a full-time job with little reward.

Bear in mind that the survivor has suffered a traumatic brain injury and will not always have control of their emotions. They are frustrated, by not being able to do what once came to them naturally and lack the control to express **Emotional intelligence** (otherwise known as **emotional quotient** or **EQ**); instead, they come over as being rude and abrupt, which can be degrading at times.

Caregivers need to look after their own health by taking time out for themselves and spending it in a place that is their go-to zone when things get tough. They need to learn when to ask others for help, even if it's only for a few hours or a day.

A burnt-out caregiver is of no use to anyone, including themselves.

Frustration Vs Aggression

The unexpected lifestyle changes can lead to numerous frustrating situations, especially with the sudden onset of a disability. To the outside world, these frustrations may be perceived as anger tantrums.

Misconstruing frustration with anger is understandable to the untrained eye. So, before retaliating and jumping to conclusions, place yourself in the shoes of the survivor and try to see things from their perspective.

For example, they might be trying to accomplish something as simple as opening a coffee jar. To the abled individual, this may seem like a simple task, but to them, attempting it with only one hand can prove to be highly frustrating.

Before being judgemental, try things for yourself and see life from their point of view.

Start by tying one hand behind your back and spend the remainder of the day like that. You might be surprised to discover just how difficult it is to do things with only one hand. Maybe then you will better understand what they are going through daily. Learn to identify those frustrating situations before they occur.

While coming to terms with their deficits, anticipate when they cannot do something and offer to help. Even better, where possible, move things around so they can do it themselves; after all, the best way to retrain the brain is to let them try things for themselves.

Rehabilitation is a long and tedious road. By continuously doing everything for them, they will only learn to become dependent on you and stop trying to do things independently.

Patience is a virtue. Retaliating to their frustrations with anger will only push them over the edge, stirring up a whirlwind of unnecessary emotions.

Instead, please take a deep breath and remember that survivors are often not in control of their actions.

Neuroplasticity

Neuro refers to the brain and **plasticity** to its pliability. Neuroplasticity is the pliability of the brain to reorganise itself throughout the life of the individual.

A survivor's family may encounter an incurious attitude from the medical staff, judiciously believing that survivors have two years to regain as much mobility as possible, after which there is no more hope. Such a carefree attitude and primitive belief of yesteryear are perhaps why survivors and their families give up all hope after such a short period of only a couple of years.

The reality is that the brain, with its neuroplasticity, keeps learning over the survivor's lifespan. With the brain continually trying to mend itself, recovery is possible many years after the initial trauma.

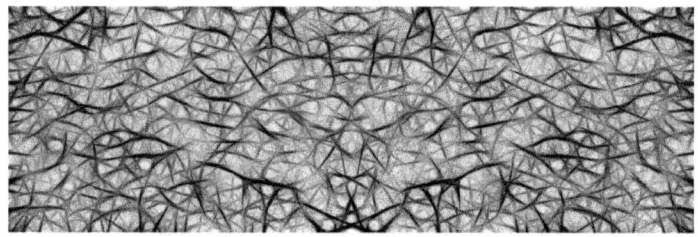

Loneliness

Such adversity has a way of filtering out your true friends from the seasonal ones, ignorance being the principal culprit.

People do not know how to react to such adversity. What

are they supposed to say, and how do they react?

Human nature is to avoid such confrontations, and so they would rather go out of their way to elude any such encounters.

Sadly, such evasions are not unique to friends. Family can also get caught up in this trap of ignorance, isolating the survivor in the process.

Secluded from friends and family, the situation can rapidly spiral out of control, resulting in loneliness and depression.

Depression

Depression is expected and easily recognisable after a Traumatic Brain Injury.

A change in mood or an aversion to activities is a typical sign of depression.

Survivors and their families can expect apathy from trauma to the brain. Fortunately, with modern medicine, one can take medication to control depression. One should not wait, before seeking out medical help.

Caregivers should not take any talk of suicide lightly, and urgent professional intervention should be sought.

The deficits brought on by the trauma may cause the survivor to become dependent on others. Their sudden loss of independence can leave them feeling despondent, and they may even start to believe that the world would be a better place without them.

Such inconsolable thoughts should not be taken lightly.

If neglected, the situation could rapidly spiral out of control.

Therefore, it is of paramount importance that they talk to an experienced professional trained in dealing with such circumstances, an independent third party who is detached from the patient's situation—someone who can take their hand and walk them through this taxing period.

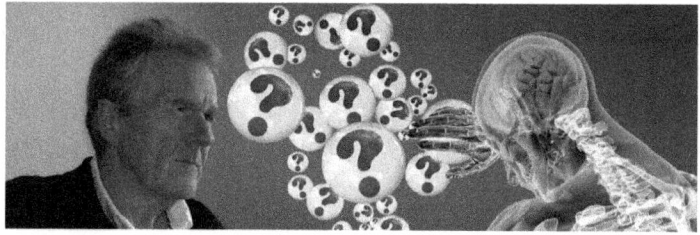

Despite what we may expect of ourselves, we are all only human. No one expects us to be equipped to handle every curveball life throws at us on our own.

Family and friends, who have stuck around, need to reassure the survivor that they love and care for them dearly. Please encourage them by letting them know that their health and safety are of utmost concern to you. It is also of paramount importance that you offer as much emotional reassurance as you can.

Anxiety

After being cooped up and isolated from society for such a long time, while in hospital, rehab and at home. The anxiety will be overwhelming the first time the survivor returns to the community, which, incidentally, may only be a trip to the corner store. The survivor might be anxious and self-conscious about their appearance, feeling that everybody is staring at them.

Reassure them that this is not the case.

To avoid such situations, they may choose to remain

isolated in the comfort of their home.

Habitually, people are curious to find out more about what happened to a physically impaired person but are ignorant of approaching the subject.

Rather than getting angry at their ignorance. Become the educator and enlighten them, so that they may have a better understanding of what you are going through. Let them walk away feeling wiser.

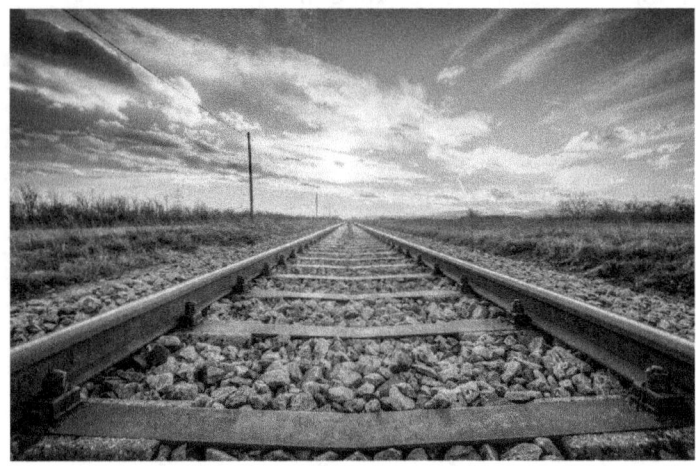

The way you see things

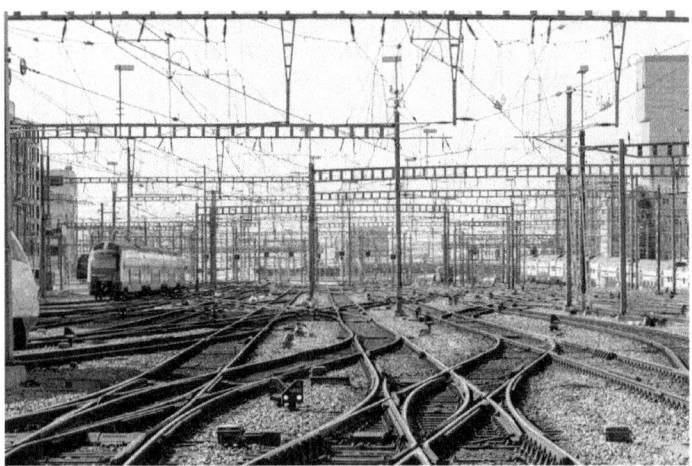

The way a survivor sees things

Remember, survivors have been through something that they have no idea about. Instead of feeling self-conscious, hold your head up high, and be proud of who you are; you are a survivor! Not many people can claim that, and no one can take that title away from you.

The good news is that the more you get out of the home, the more comfortable you will become and the less anxious you will begin to feel. Start with baby steps and gradually increase your exposure to crowds.

When the author initially went out into public, he anxiously paused if a crowd was approaching and waited for them to pass before moving on. The more exposure he got to the masses, the easier it got.

Exposure does heal anxiety.

Dressing And Grooming

Two of life's daily activities are to dress and groom oneself. Attempting these tasks after a brain injury can be more challenging than initially anticipated. With a caregiver to assist, the task will be substantially simplified. Doing it on your own is another story, for another day.

Whether you have assistance or not, remember to always lead with your weak side. In other words, when putting on a shirt, start by inserting your weak arm into the sleeve, followed by your stronger arm.

Do the same with your trousers. Putting on trousers by yourself, with a foot that will not come to the party, is much like trying to put on trousers with your sneakers on, for an abled person.

When it comes to shoes, help will be required until they have enough strength in the leg muscles to lift their foot. In the beginning, it is easier to use shoes with Velcro straps as tying shoelaces with one hand, although possible, is an art on its own. Over time and with some help from their therapist, the survivor will learn some tricks to achieve this. An alternative is to replace the laces with a silicon lacing system. Converting your lace-up shoes to slip on.

Grooming may prove challenging initially, significantly so if their dominant side was affected, but in time, they will learn new tricks, and when they do so, it will get easier. Refrain from letting survivors use any razors or sharp objects on their own.

Medication And Its Side Effects

Following a traumatic Brain Injury, the survivor may find that they have been prescribed more medications

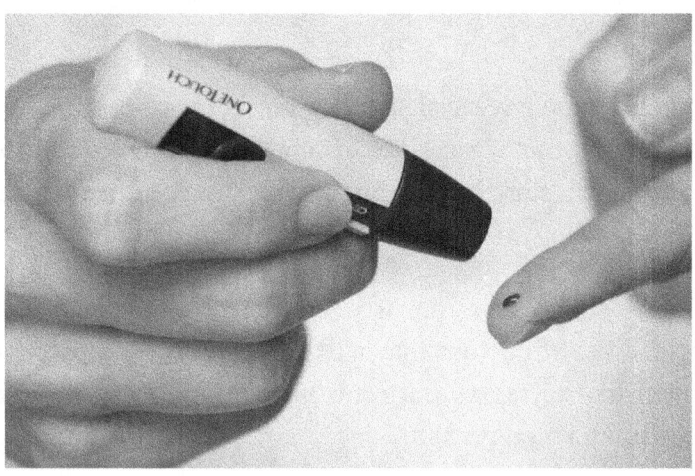

than they are used to.

These medicines come with a compilation of side effects. Sadly, these side effects can be more unpleasant than they need to be.

For some reason, it may be difficult for the survivor's family to convince the medical staff to take them as seriously as they should. Family members and caregivers alike need to *familiarise themselves* with all the medications and their side effects.

With so many side effects, if the survivor begins to act out of character, urgently seek medical assistance and advise them on what is transpiring.

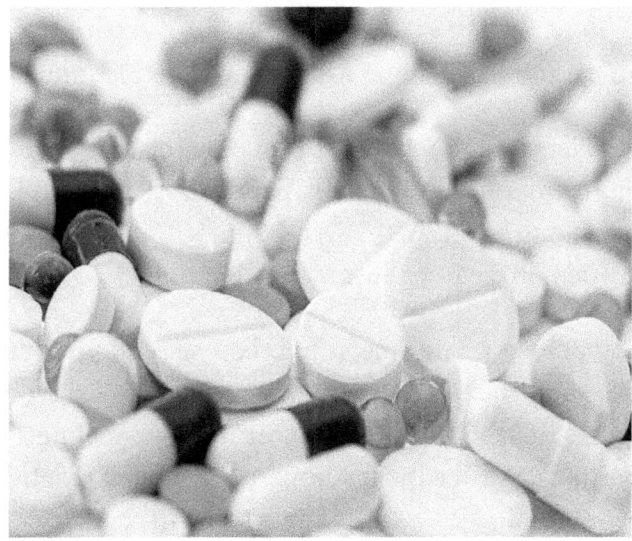

You are the survivor's advocate. *Don't let the Doctor off the hook* until they have answered all your questions and have suggested some concrete solutions.

Your only weapon is loads of questions.

Ask them,
'What can we do about…'
or
'Isn't there a different medication that…'

INTIMACY AFTER A TBI

Intimacy and sex after TBI have always been contentious and avoided at all costs. Intimacy may still be possible depending on where in the brain the injury occurred and its severity.

BEFORE ENGAGING IN ANY INTIMACY, PLEASE CLEAR THIS WITH YOUR DOCTOR.

Sex can be just as fulfilling as it was before the injury.

However, engaging in exotic sexual positions may prove to be more arduous, hindered by paralysis. Penetration is not everything, and with a little bit of imagination, foreplay can prove to be just as exhilarating.

Intimacy does not only mean intercourse, and you may want to start the foreplay by kissing, caressing and massaging. Start slowly, communicate your feelings to your partner, and let them know about your anxieties. With communication, together, you will be able to experiment and discover comfortable positions that will satisfy both your needs.

A Positive Mind Yields Positive Results

Don't expect everything to be okay straight away.

Recovery is a deliberate process that requires arduous hours of repetition. Patience and perseverance are the keys to effective rehabilitation.

Motivating the survivor as much as possible will get them moving, but it's their determination to get better that will keep them going. Don't ever give up.

Technology is advancing at such a rampant pace, and scientists are continually finding new ways to help survivors recover from their harrowing ordeal.

Even the toughest of the tough, the "well-adjusted" survivor who thinks they are doing well, will have some tough days.

Delayed reactions are par to recovery.

Many survivors steel themselves to their loss and feel strong. That is until the slightest whisper of hope. It will cause a seasoned survivor's eyes to well up with tears of joy. That twitch of hope is enough to instil confidence. Hang in there for as long as it takes.

As their caregiver, re-enforce how proud you are of them – over and over again, session after session, year after year. Never give up hope. The more love and affection they receive, the more determined they will be to recover! Recovery is a slooooooooow and tedious process; I am talking glacial speed, so don't expect overnight miracles.

Every action begins with the tiniest of twitches. The recovery process may slow down with time, but it will only stop when they, and only they, decide to give up.

Never give up, and remember that *no is never an option*.

CHAPTER SIX

In-patient rehabilitation

What Is In-House Rehabilitation?

In-house rehabilitation is also known as inpatient rehabilitation or acute rehabilitation.

The aim of inpatient rehabilitation is to return patients safely to their home environment. Such rehabilitation may be part of a larger hospital group or a private or government facility.

Patients usually remain in these facilities for about two or three weeks.

During their stay, they participate in an intensive, well-coordinated rehabilitation program.

Rehabilitation is intense during this period, as the recovery process is at its peak.

In-house rehabilitation facilities are not miracle centres, and recovery does not end when they leave. Recovering from a TBI is ongoing and can continue for the remainder of the survivor's life but at a much slower rate.

It was once thought that the brain stopped healing after a year or two, but this has been proven wrong.

Through a process known as neuroplasticity, the brain learns and rewires itself for the remainder of the patients' lives.

In-house rehabilitation is only the beginning. The first

few months are when the most rehabilitation is observed. After that, it begins to slow down but never stops. To take advantage of this limited window period, inpatient therapy is intensive and consists of all the necessary therapy to get the patient back home again. Therapy consists of Physiotherapy, Occupational therapy and Speech therapy. A Psychologist might be necessary to help with the emotional side of the injury.

In-house rehabilitation may also contain other forms of therapy that are deemed necessary, such as recreational therapy, art, and music.

Is It Important?

The first three months following a TBI are the most important for recovery. This is when patients will see the most improvement. During this time, patients will enter and complete a two to three week inpatient rehabilitation program, after which they will move on to an outpatient therapy program.

On entering an in-house facility, the patient's family needs to realise that their loved one has undergone a significant change in life. The family will need to realise that the TBI survivor may have been taken back in time as far as their independence. They may no longer be able to do certain things for themselves and will need help. They will need to relearn these tasks if they ever want to regain some independence.

During therapy at an in-house facility, they will be taught daily living activities that most of us take for granted. Besides their daily mandatory therapy sessions, survivors will be taught how to dress and groom themselves, how to go to the bathroom on their own safely, plus much more.

In-house rehabilitation is that stepping stone to regaining some independence.

CHAPTER SEVEN

Out-patient rehabilitation

What Is Out-Patient Rehabilitation?

An outpatient facility is where patients go for continued therapy once they have completed their initial three week inpatient program. Selecting a suitable facility is of crucial importance, as therapy needs to be individualised to each patient's needs. Recovering from any brain injury is not a one-size-fits-all scenario.

Each rehabilitation program needs to be customised to the survivor's specific needs, and the therapists will need to discuss this amongst themselves and the family.

The most successful therapy comes from a team of therapists who can get together and discuss the progress and future needs of the patient. The teams need to communicate with the family and provide them with regular progress updates.

Depending on the inpatient facility the patient was at, they might also offer an outpatient program. If this is the case, the patient could continue with them but as an outpatient. If the facility does not provide this service, the patient family would have to look for an independent outpatient facility.

Searching for the correct facilities may involve finding a rehab with everything under one roof or individual therapists located in different practices.

The family must ensure that the therapists are neuro trained if going the latter route.

Is It Important?

After a brief period of intense and exhausting in-patient rehabilitation, survivors are discharged from the safe compound of the in-house facility and released back into a cruel and unforgiving society.

Formal outpatient rehabilitation is critical for survivors to regain as much independence and confidence as possible. The time and money spent on proper outpatient rehabilitation are precious, so selecting a suitable facility is critical.

Survivors might not be able to do exactly what they did before the TBI, and rehabilitation is not a miracle cure.

Rehab cannot repair damaged tissue in the brain. However, through a process known as neuroplasticity, the brain has the amazing ability to rewire itself, allowing the neurons (nerve cells) in the brain to compensate for the injury by adjusting their activities in response to the new changes in their environment.

CHAPTER EIGHT

Therapy

Physiotherapy

Physical therapy or physiotherapy (often abbreviated to PT) is a form of rehabilitation where physical intervention to an injured area is required to encourage mobility and function to re-establish quality of life.

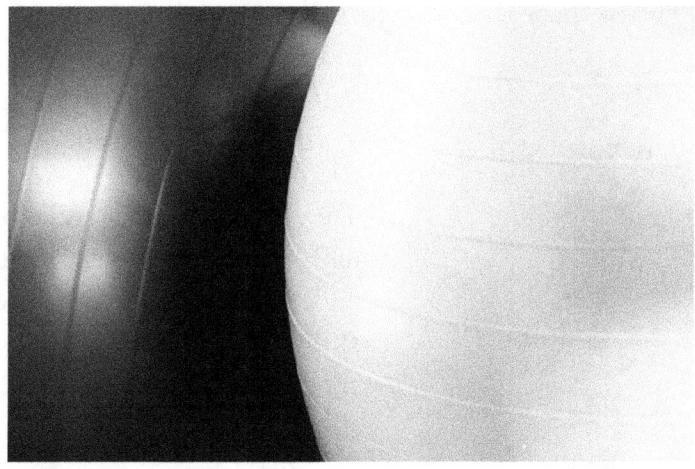

For TBI survivors, physiotherapists focus on the lower limbs to regain their balance and walking ability.

The lower limbs are also usually the first to respond to any therapy.

Occupational Therapy

Occupational Therapy (OT), on the other hand, focuses on the upper limb, the shoulder, arm and hand. The OT works on recovering and maintaining skills used in daily living and work activities.

OT's deal with people who have physical, mental or cognitive disorders. They attempt to restore a patient's

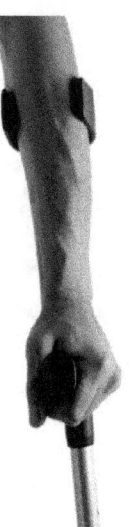

independence by identifying and eliminating environmental barriers.

They help patients to relearn daily skills involving hand and arm movements. These skills include bathing, tying shoelaces or buttoning one's shirt.

OTs also address cognitive issues and safety in the home.

They help survivors address returning-to-work issues if that is a viable option.

An occupational therapist's involvement centres on increasing participation and performance in daily

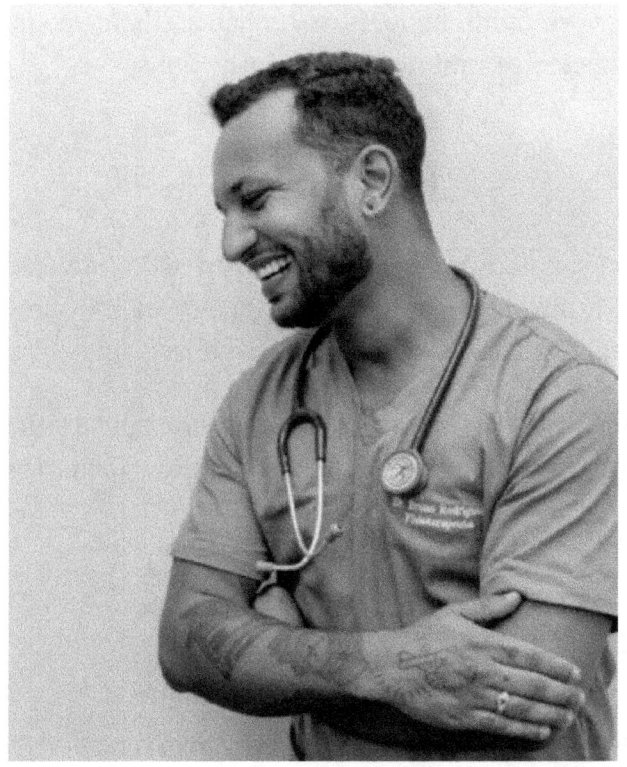

activities by adapting the environment and modifying the task to teach the survivor and their family the necessary skills.

The upper limb, however, is usually slow to respond to therapy.

Speech Therapy

Speech and vocational Therapists improve patients

language skills and, where necessary, their ability to swallow.

They work with patients to enhance their memory, thinking and communication imperfections.

Biokinetics

Biokinetists are exercise specialists who increase a patient's physical condition and quality of life through physical evaluations and healthy exercise habits.

Biokinetics is a step up from physiotherapy. Both are important, and the survivor needs to follow the process.

There are no shortcuts to recovering from a TBI.

Neuropsychologist

Is there a difference between a clinical psychologist and a neuropsychologist?

Yes, most definitely, a clinical psychologist focuses more on the patient's emotional side whereas a neuropsychologist focuses on the patient's cognitive processes, neurobehavioral and brain disorders.

A neuropsychologist is a professional trained in evaluating disorders associated with neurological trauma.

Being detached from the situation, they are able to approach the problem with a clear mind. They are able to assess whether the patients thinking skills are emotional or neurobehavioral.

Social Worker

Social workers help connect patients to financial resources and plan for their new living arrangements if necessary.

They educate patients and their families on entitlements, community resources, and health insurance coverage.

They are directed toward helping patients, and their families adjust to living with a disability. Where possible, they facilitate the patient's return to the community at the highest possible functional, social and economic level.

CHAPTER NINE

Support groups

What Are Support Groups

Support groups provide survivors, their families and caregivers a space to talk freely about their challenges and issues without being judged. Sharing stories with others on a similar plight can give one a sense of empowerment and control, which can reduce stress and depression. Participants may be surprised to discover just how much they have in common with each other and that they are not alone on this lonely ambivalent journey.

One of the concerns to an already tricky recovery is social isolation. Humans by nature are social animals; who need plenty of interaction with one another to thrive. But for survivors who may have a wide range of disabilities, social contact and interaction can be challenging - even when their families are close at hand. Support groups break the isolation cycle and provide a safe haven to interact with others.

Mental health professionals understand that support groups effectively cope with the stresses, changes and challenges of going through a significant life-altering event, like Traumatic Brain Injury.

Not everyone copes with a neurological impairment in the same way. A support group is a great way to get to know other survivors and learn how they deal with their situation. The open, non-judgemental nature of a support group is one of the best ways to feel that they are not alone.

Benefits Of A Support Group

Support groups have numerous benefits which, include:

- Countering loneliness and isolation.
- Providing a non-judgmental, compassionate space to talk about one's feelings.
- They give members a way to improve their coping skills and help them to adjust to their new situation.
- Reducing stress, anxiety, depression, and fatigue.
- Participants have access to information about doctors, treatments, and other resources in their community that they may not have known about.
- They help participants to make new friends who share their situation.
- Help answer questions that doctors can't.

A strong support system is the backbone of any successful rehabilitation.

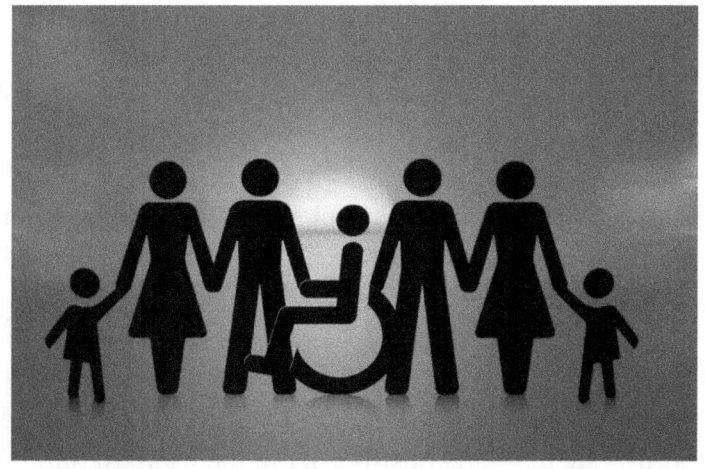

Often, survivors and their families do not know where to find assistance or whom to turn to for help. Instead of bottling things up, survivors must have the opportunity to talk about how they feel. Support is imperative to recovery and overcoming these barriers that prevent them from getting out and participating.

They provide a comfortable environment to learn, share stories, gain encouragement and develop new friendships.

Socialising with others going through a similar plight has proven to be a great support system.

Should Caregivers Attend Support Groups?

Support groups are just as important for caregivers as

they are for survivors.

Caregivers can rapidly find themselves being absorbed into the life of the survivor.

A support group provides a place for them to vent and will help them to find an even balance between caregiving and time out.

Engaging in an active social life and relationships with friends and family is vitally important to a caregiver, as it allows them to feel positive about themselves. Support groups are a perfect place to make new friends.

A burnt-out caregiver is of no use to anyone.

CHAPTER TEN

Stages of grief

5 Stages Of Grief

A positive mindset is vital for a productive recovery, coupled with countless hours of repetitive therapy.

Traumatic Brain Injury is a family affliction that does not only affect the survivor. It might signify the harsh reality of the 'death' of the person you once knew and loved so dearly and the re-birth of a 'new' survivor in their place.

Learn to accept the survivor for whom they have become. Their change in conduct could prove to be extremely tough and emotional for everyone. Therefore, a grieving period is required, which will lead you through various emotional stages, from denial to anger, bargaining, depression, and finally onto acceptance.

These steps do not necessarily happen in this order and can vary from person to person.

Denial

Denial is not a river in Africa; it is the start of the grieving process. It can leave a person feeling numb, disorientated and overwhelmed by what has just happened.

It helps people survive and get through the trauma during a stage where the world becomes meaningless and overwhelming. Life as you know it suddenly makes no sense, and you begin to wonder how you will ever continue living.

In the early days following the trauma, an overpowering feeling of numbness is expected. Some family and friends may find it hard to come to terms with what happened and will be in disbelief. They might question how this could have happened in the first place and will carry on as though nothing had happened.

Denial is nature's way of allowing people to deal with the grief, and it will enable you to take on as much as you can handle at a time. Questions about what the future may hold is a lot of hypothetical information to process. Denial is a way of slowing down this process and taking the person through it, one step at a time.

Once you come to terms with the reality of the present, you will begin to question yourself. Unknowingly you are beginning the healing process. You will gradually become stronger, and the feelings of denial will begin to subside.

Anger

Anger is a common occurrence amongst TBI survivors. Suddenly and without warning, they find themselves wallowing in a pool of uncertainty.

The sudden lifestyle change could lead to anger outbursts that may be redirected towards anybody in close proximity. It may be towards anyone they feel they could spread the blame onto for their situation.

The sudden loss of independence is devastating, and trying to accept the deficits can be just as overwhelming.

Bargaining And Negotiating

Bargaining or negotiating is when you find yourself asking many questions.

Questions such as:

'What if I had only' and wondering what you could have done differently,

'If only I could have one more chance' or 'If only I had done..... differently.'

Attempting to negotiate with your loss is an all too familiar scenario. Coming to terms with what has just happened to you is tough.

Depression

Depression is the most easily recognisable sign and is commonly expected with TBI survivors. Regrettably, it does not only affect the survivor; instead, it touches all who are close to them.

Each person will be affected to a different degree. Those not directly affected may not realise its impact on the family and what they are going through. They might even expect them to snap out of this stage of depression and sadness and get on with their lives, which is easier said than done.

The family have just 'lost' a loved one, someone they loved so dearly. They need to mourn their loss and accept the new survivor who has emerged in their place. Life has just taken a drastic turn, and their future is now filled with ambiguity and uncertainty.

No one can handle such adversity on their own and will need to seek professional help, someone they can talk to freely about what they are going through. Seeking out professional help in light of what has happened is highly recommended for all who are dear to the survivor.

A neuropsychologist is detached from the situation and trained to assist in such trying times. Having just been through a traumatic experience, there is nothing that can prepare one for the tsunami of emotional upsurges they are about to encounter.

With the road ahead having been tainted with so much ambiguity, you need the assistance of someone with a clear head. Someone you can talk to who can guide you through this upsurge.

Acceptance

Coming to terms with the reality of being or being a caregiver to a TBI survivor is one of the most challenging stages to acknowledge.

Admitting to a future filled with deficits and uncertainties is no easy task. Acknowledging that you might depend on others for basic daily living chores is no easy task.

Chores they once took for granted, and that they could do with their eyes shut, may suddenly have become mammoth undertakings requiring the assistance of a Caregiver. Tasks like dressing, cooking or getting around –might require the services of a caregiver and driver.

Personal hygiene might necessitate assistance as well.

Try and understand what the survivor is going through. They might find themselves powerless and resemble a child trapped in an adult's body. They may need the assistance of someone to help them bathe or even wash up after having gone to the bathroom.

If you, as a Caregiver, find this humiliating, consider the humiliation that they are plagued with. They never asked to be placed in such a predicament. The Brain Injury has put them there.

The survivor is now faced with uncertainties that they were never prepared for, be they of a physical or cognitive in nature. They might find themselves asking you many questions.

Don't be intimidated by the numerous questions they might ask – no one expects you to be a medical expert and have all the answers. You are there to act as a sounding board for them, someone who will listen without judging. Let them bounce their thoughts and fears off you. Remember always to remain positive and reassure them that you will be with them, one hundred per cent of the way. Listen to their fears and emotional anxieties; after all, they have been through a traumatic rollercoaster.

Keep offering as much emotional reassurance as you can.

CHAPTER ELEVEN

Hyperbaric Oxygen Therapy (HBOT)

What Is Hyperbaric Oxygen Therapy

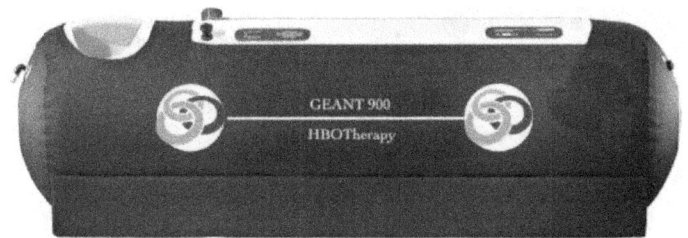

Before getting started, we need to understand the meaning of Atmospheric and Hyperbaric pressure.

Atmospheric pressure is the force exerted on a surface from a column of air above it due to the Earth's gravitational pull.

Hyperbaric pressure is an operating pressure greater than normal atmospheric pressure.

Hence, HyperBaric Oxygen Therapy (HBOT) is the administering of oxygen under increased pressure.

Hyperbaric Oxygen Therapy is a medical procedure whereby the body is enclosed in a full-bodied chamber and exposed to increased oxygen levels while under pressure greater than atmospheric pressure (the outside pressure).

It is a painless non-evasive procedure.

Under normal circumstances, the atmospheric pressure exerted on the body at sea level is one atmosphere (ATA).

As we ascend to altitude, the pressure begins to decrease, increasing the size of the individual gas molecules.

When we descend, the opposite happens, and the pressure increases, reducing the size of the individual gas molecules.

How Does It Work?

Hyperbaric Oxygen Therapy (HBOT) works by increasing the pressure in a controlled environment (an enclosed chamber) and delivering increased amounts of oxygen to the patient.

Every day, the air we breathe comprises 21% oxygen, 78% nitrogen, and 1% inert gases.

Under normal circumstances, our bodies can mend themselves using the oxygen levels found in the air. However, certain conditions require additional oxygen.

This is where HBOT comes in. During Hyperbaric Oxygen Therapy, the pressure inside the chamber is gradually increased to above atmospheric pressure (outside pressure), and the breathing of pure oxygen commences. Because the body is exposed to increased pressure, the oxygen molecules are also under pressure and are smaller in size. Therefore, significant amounts of oxygen can be dissolved into the hard-to-reach blood plasma, cerebrospinal fluid (the fluid surrounding the brain and spinal cord), lymph, bone, and other body fluids.

Oxygen saturates the body and enhances the functioning of the white blood cells, which form part of the immune system that protects the body against infectious disease and foreign invaders—promoting the body's ability to aid in self-healing.

Not only does the increased oxygen levels reduce swelling and inflammation, but it also promotes the growth of new blood vessels into the affected areas with reduced circulation.

Increasing the Oxygen levels in damaged tissues allows the body's natural healing mechanisms to function more effectively, even when the blood supply has been compromised.

With the aid of HBOT, damaged tissues can receive oxygen via other body fluids from surrounding areas, in addition to stimulating the release of stem cells.

Hyperbaric Oxygen Therapy is particularly effective in delivering increased oxygen to deep tissue infections with a poor blood supply.

Regular exposure to oxygen under pressure prompts and speeds up the body's natural healing process of wounds.

You may be asking why you have to use HBOT; surely

an increase in oxygen would do the same thing?

You would be wrong. Remember that the individual gas molecules will decrease in size as we increase the pressure. This includes the oxygen molecules as well. Swelling and inflammation cause the blood vessels in the compromised tissue to constrict, reducing the flow of oxygenated blood to the wound.

Under pressure (HBOT), the body can carry those smaller oxygen molecules dissolved into the blood plasma, cerebrospinal fluid, lymph, bone, and other body fluids to the compromised tissue, increasing oxygen supply and facilitating the healing process.

HBOT IS BASED ON TWO PARTIAL PRESSURE LAWS

Henry's Law and **Dalton's Law.**

- **Henry's Law** states that "At a constant temperature, the amount of a given gas that dissolves in a given type and volume of liquid is directly proportional to the partial pressure of that gas in equilibrium with that liquid.

  In other words, at a constant temperature, as the pressure increases on a liquid, the liquid will hold more gas molecules.

This theory can easily be seen in everyday use, i.e., soda drinks.

- **SODA EFFECT**: Soda is essentially syrup and water. Under normal conditions (one ATA), the pressure on the liquid is in equilibrium with the atmospheric pressure. By increasing the pressure in an enclosed container, we can dissolve carbon dioxide into the liquid and keep it there whilst under pressure. Once the container has been opened, the sudden release in pressure will cause the carbon dioxide to come out of suspension in an attempt to reach equilibrium with the outside atmospheric pressure. This gives us the fizziness we all enjoy in our Sodas.

Once equilibrium has been reached, we refer to the soda as being flat.

- **Dalton's Law of** Partial Pressure states "that in a mixture of non-reacting gases, the total pressure exerted is equal to the sum of the partial pressures of the individual gases".

  In other words, the total pressure is made up of the sum of all the individual gases under pressure.

  $$i.e.: P_{Total} = P_1 + P_2 \ldots\ldots + P_n.$$

Understanding HBOT

Red blood cells are limited to the amount of oxygen that can bind with the haemoglobin (the protein in red blood cells). The plasma (the clear yellowish fluid portion of blood) only carries about 3% of the oxygen concentration.

Placing a patient into a hyperbaric environment at pressures greater than atmospheric pressure and combined with an increased oxygen partial pressure allows the body to dissolve more of the smaller oxygen molecules into its blood cells, blood plasma, cerebral-spinal fluid, bone and other body fluids.

These oxygen-enriched, saturated fluids are then delivered to all of the body's cells, tissues, and fluids in higher than normal concentrations, which dramatically accelerates the healing process.

Portable hyperbaric chambers are typically pressurised to 1.3 ATA, being about 0.3 ATA above the outside atmospheric pressure. I say about because this will vary with altitude.

1,3 ATA is equivalent to approximately the same pressure you would experience while diving down to the bottom of a swimming pool in the deep end.

The increased oxygen concentration enhances the function of the white blood cells, boosting the immune system and promoting the body's ability to aid in self-healing.

Not only does the increased pressure and oxygen levels reduce inflammation and swelling, but it also promotes the growth of new blood vessels into the affected area.

Increasing oxygen levels into damaged tissues allows the body's natural healing mechanisms to function more effectively, even with a compromised blood supply. Damaged tissues can now receive oxygen via the blood plasma and other body fluids from surrounding areas.

Hyperbaric Oxygen Therapy is particularly effective in delivering increased amounts of oxygen to wounds with poor blood flow or injured tissue that is swollen. Daily exposure to these increased amounts of oxygen enables the body to speed up the healing process of the wound.

What Pressure Is Used?

When hyperbaric therapy was first used, higher pressures of 2-4 ATA of pressure and 100% oxygen were used.

The world of hyperbaric medicine has since realised that lower pressures (1.3 ATA as in the portable chambers approved by the FDA for use in the home and 1.3-1.5 ATA in larger hospital and clinic-based chambers) with less oxygen (often 21 to 40%) seem to have excellent effects on multiple systems of our bodies.

In particular, lower pressure appears to be more beneficial for the injured brain than higher pressure.

How Long Are Treatments?

Treatments may also be referred to as dives and are usually 60-90 minutes per session, 5-7 times per week.

Daily treatments are required to achieve the best benefits.

Are There Any Side Effects?

Hyperbaric Oxygen Therapy is a painless and non-evasive procedure with no side effects.

However, some people may feel tired after a treatment. Others may experience popping in their ears. Few may have minor changes in vision, but these changes are temporary.

What Will I Experience?

A patient will experience a change in pressure in their ears when the chamber begins to pressurise. Similar to that felt on an aeroplane when it begins its descent.

Usually, swallowing or yawning will alleviate any discomfort. You can also pinch your nose and gently blow. Any of these methods will equalise the pressure in your ears with the chamber's ambient pressure.

At the end of each session, the chamber pressure is reduced, returning it to the outside ambient pressure.

During this stage, the ears will automatically equalise themselves.

What Is The Doughnut Effect?

Injured tissue resembles a doughnut. The hollow, middle portion of the doughnut is the traumatised area. This tissue is the area directly affected by the trauma—dead tissue in the case of a brain injury. Nothing can be done to revive this dead tissue.

This dead tissue is encircled by inflamed, compromised tissue, forming a doughnut shape around the trauma, hence the name. This impaired tissue is not dead but

The Doughnut Effect

Impaired
Tissue

Dead
Tissue

Inflamed, compromised tissue

rather inflamed, constricting the blood vessels in its path and restricting oxygen flow.

When placing a patient into a hyperbaric chamber and getting them to breathe oxygen while at pressure, it causes the oxygen molecules to constrict in size, allowing them to penetrate the compromised tissue.

The combination of the hyperbaric environment and the increased oxygen partial pressure allows the body to dissolve more oxygen into its blood cells, blood plasma, cerebral-spinal fluid, bone and other body fluids.

This increase in oxygen concentration enhances the function of the white blood cells, stimulating the immune system and *promoting* the body's ability to heal itself.

These smaller oxygen molecules can now reach the compromised tissue at increased pressures and in higher concentrations. The increased absorption promotes the growth of new blood vessels into the affected area, helping to reduce inflammation.

Increasing oxygen levels into the damaged tissue allows the body's natural healing mechanisms to function more effectively, even with a compromised blood supply. Damaged tissues can now receive oxygen, initiating the healing process.

CHAPTER TWELVE

Electrical Stimulation

Electrical Muscle Stimulation (EMS)

EMS uses an electrical current produced by a battery-operated device to stimulate muscle movement. The unit is connected to the skin by two or more electrodes placed strategically on the muscle. With one being positive and the other negative, current passing between the two electrodes causes the muscles to be stimulated

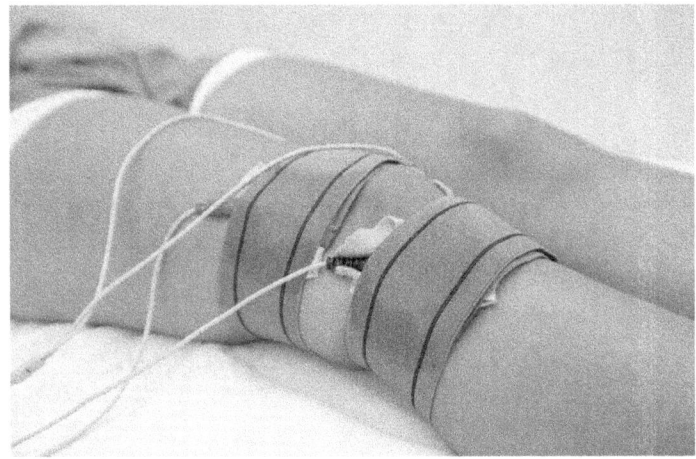

The operator can vary the intensity of the electrical current, and the device can be programmed for various cycles. Each cycle is programmed to achieve a different result.

Transcutaneous Electrical Nerve Sti mulation (TENS)

TENS units also use an electrical current produced by a battery-operated device to stimulate the nerves for therapeutic purposes.
Transcutaneous Electrical Nerve Stimulation units
cover the complete range of transcutaneously applied currents used for nerve stimulation.

TENS is used to describe the kind of pulses produced by these portable stimulators to treat pain. The unit has two or more electrodes, which are strategically connected to the skin, through which current is passed.

Functional Electrical Stimulation

(FES)

Functional Electrical Stimulation is used during daily practical activities, the most common being dorsiflexion.

Dorsiflexion is the backwards movement of the front part of the foot and its digits. It is a crucial action required while walking. Dorsiflexion allows the front section of the foot to lift, allowing the foot to strike the ground on its return in the accustomed heel-to-toe action, offering stability with each step. A movement we all take for granted, and no one thinks about it when they walk or run; it is something that happens automatically. That is, until you lose the luxury and then with every step you take, it becomes your only thought.

A traumatic brain or nerve injury could result in you losing this fundamental function, resulting in gait abnormality from the foot drop. Damage to the fibular nerve causes this. Deprived of such an essential luxury, your foot then begins to droop, and the toes drag over the ground. Providing you with the unique ability to trip over air.

When you can no longer walk in a heel-to-toe manner, the drooping foot begins to slap itself onto the ground in one movement. Besides being painful, the hanging foot causes you to become very unstable on your feet.

Foot drop is responsible for some debilitating falls. To prevent tripping, patients have had to adjust their walking gait in a desperate attempt to be mobile. They have resorted to elevating their hip and circumducting the weak leg as they walk. Circumduction is a hemiplegic gait in which the leg is stiff with no flexion at the knee and ankle. With each step, the survivor rotates the leg away from the body and then back in towards it again, forming a semi-circle with each step. Such a walking gait only leads to further complications over time.

The alternative has always been to wear an ankle-foot Orthosis (AFO) to lift the flaccid foot while supporting the ankle. Not only do AFO's extend from below the knee, but they are also cumbersome and uncomfortable to wear.

Today, functional electrical stimulation (FES) units are available due to modern technology. They allow survivors to walk with a more 'natural' gait, as they help stimulate the appropriate nerves and muscles when walking.

Once programmed to your needs, the FES works with each step you take. Depending on the unit, they either have a built-in tilt sensor or a heel switch that triggers the unit every time you step on it, sending an electrical pulse to activate the nerves. Having stimulated the peroneal nerve, the front of the foot lifts and tilts backwards, allowing the survivor to walk with a more natural gait.

CHAPTER THIRTEEN

Terminology

Easy Reference

Adult Diaper - A diaper made to be worn by adults

Ankle Foot Orthosis (AFO) - A brace used to support the foot and ankle

Anxiety - Nervous behaviour; a state of uneasiness

Aqua Therapy - Exercises performed in water

Atrial Fibrillation - An irregular heartbeat

Ageusia - An impaired sense of taste

Agnosia - The inability to recognise an object by touch alone

Agraphia - Struggle in writing or drawing

Alexia - Inability to read

Amnesia - Loss of memory

Aneurysm - The swelling of a blood vessel that may rupture and bleed, causing a stroke

Angioplasty - A procedure to improve blood flow by stretching narrowed coronary artery

Aphagia - The inability to swallow

Aphasia - A partial or total loss of the ability to articulate ideas or comprehend spoken or written language, resulting from damage to the brain caused by the stroke

Apathy - A lack of feeling, emotion and interest

Apraxia - Struggle to coordinate movement or speech

Ataxia - Loss of muscle function

Atheroma - A build-up of fatty deposits in blood vessels that restrict blood flow

Atherosclerosis - A build-up of cholesterol, fats and other substances in and on the artery walls

Arteriovenous Malformation (AVM) - An abnormal structure of arteries and veins within the brain that runs the risk of a haemorrhage

Atrial Fibrillation (AFib) - An irregular, often rapid heart rate that usually causes poor blood flow

Blood Pressure - Pressure of blood inside the arteries

Blood thinners - Medication used to thin blood

Botox - A neurotoxic protein used to ease high tone temporarily

Brain attack - A new term for a stroke

Brainstem - Posterior part of the brain and is a continuation of the spinal cord, responsible for basic life functions

Caregiver - An individual who helps another with an impairment with their Activities of Daily Living (ADL)

Carotid Arteries - Blood vessels that supply oxygenated blood to the brain and neck

Carotid Doppler - Ultrasound of the arteries in the neck to check for blockages

Carotid Endarterectomy - A procedure to clear a blockage from a Carotid Artery

CAT Scan - Computerised Axial Tomography Scan, a two-dimensional scan used to look at sections of the body in detail

Central Stroke Pain (Central Pain Syndrome) - A mixture of sensational pain that occurs after a stroke due to damage in the thalamus area of the brain. These sensations include burning brought on by hot and cold.

Cerebrospinal fluid (CSF) - A clear, colourless that surrounds the brain and spinal cord.

Cerebrovascular Disease - A group of conditions that affect blood flow and the blood vessels in the brain

Cerebral Haemorrhage - Medical term for a bleed in the brain

Cholesterol - Fatty deposits in the arteries

Clonus - A series of involuntary rhythmic muscle contractions and relaxations

Cognitive Impairment - When a person has difficulty remembering, learning, concentrating or making decisions that affect their everyday life.

Contracture - When a joint becomes fixed in one position

Cerebrovascular Accident (CVA) - The medical term for a stroke

Deep Vein Thrombosis (DVT) - A blood clot that forms in a vein deep in the body

Depression - A low mood disorder, depressed mood

Diabetes - The build-up of glucose(sugar) in one's blood caused by the inability of the pancreas to produce enough insulin (a hormone that allows the body to absorb sugar).

Diplopia - Double vision

Dorsiflexion - The flexion or extension of the foot at the ankle. The raising of the foot where the toes are brought closer to the shin

Dysarthria - Weakness of the muscle used in speaking, making communication difficult

Dysphagia - Difficulty swallowing

Dyslexia - Difficulty reading

Dysphasia - Difficulty using and understanding language

Dysphonia - Difficulty speaking at a desired volume

Dyspraxia - Difficulty coordinating movement or speech

Eccentric Exercises - In *eccentric contraction*, the tension generated is insufficient to overcome the external load on the muscle, and the muscle fibres lengthen as they contract.

Rather than working to pull a joint in the direction of the muscle contraction, the muscle acts to decelerate the joint at the end of a movement or otherwise control the repositioning of a load.

Edema - Swelling caused by excess fluid being trapped in body tissues

Electrical Stimulation - Electrical impulses are used to stimulate muscles and contract muscles

Embolism - The lodging of an embolus, a blockage-causing piece of material, inside a blood vessel

Embolic Stroke - Occurs when a blood clot that forms elsewhere in the body breaks loose and travels to the brain.

Embolus - A clot, plaque, or other material travels through the bloodstream and creates blockages.

Emotional liability - Prone to strong feelings and sudden mood swings

EMS - Electrical Muscle Stimulation

Endothelial wall - A single layer of cells that line the inside of a blood vessel.

Feeding Tube - A medical device used to feed nutrient supplements to survivors who cannot swallow. Nutrients are supplied directly to the survivors' stomachs.

Foot drop - Is the dropping of the forefoot due to weakness of the muscle

Gait - The pattern of movement of the limbs while moving, walking

HBOT - Hyperbaric Oxygen Therapy

Hemianopia - Blindness in half the visual field in both eyes

Hemiparesis - Weakness or partial paralysis on one side of the body

Hemiplegia - Complete paralysis on one side of the body

Haemorrhage - Bleeding from a ruptured blood vessel

Haemorrhagic Stroke - Bleeding onto the brain from a ruptured blood vessel, restricting oxygenated blood flow

Haematoma - A blood clot

High Blood Pressure - Blood pressure that is too high inside the arteries

High-density lipoprotein (HDL) - AKA "good cholesterol". HDL helps move the "bad cholesterol" from the arteries back to the liver to break down and leave the body.

Hydrocephalus - Raised pressure within the skull

Hyperextension - A movement beyond normal limits

Hyperlipidemia (High Cholesterol) -Too many lipids (or fat) in the blood.

Hypertension - High blood pressure

Hypotension - Low blood pressure

Hypoxia - A state of decreased oxygen delivery to a cell

Incontinence - Loss of control of the bladder or bowel

Infarct - An area of tissue damaged by the lack of oxygen and blood

Infarction - A sudden loss of blood supply to tissue - causing the tissue to die.

Intracerebral Haemorrhage (ICH) -Bleeding into the brain tissue

Ischemic Penumbra - Areas of damaged brain tissue that still has living brain cells arranged around an area of dead brain cells that are still salvageable if reperfused.

Ischaemia - Lack of blood flow to tissues within the body

Ischaemic stroke -Blockage of a blood vessel restricting the blood flow in the brain

Lacunar Syndrome (LACS) - Medical classification of a stroke in one of the brain's smaller arteries

Lacunar Infarction - Blockage of a small artery deep in the brain resulting in a small area of damaged brain tissue.

Large Vessel Disease - Abnormalities in the large brain arteries.

Low-density lipoprotein (LDL) - Also known as the "bad cholesterol".

Locked-in Syndrome (LIS) - Locked-in Syndrome is a condition where a survivor is conscious and aware of their environment but unable to move or communicate verbally due to complete paralysis of nearly every muscle in the body; nevertheless, they are still able to move their eyes and through eye movement, communicate with the outside world

Micro haemorrhage - Small chronic brain bleeds

Mirror Therapy - Used to improve motor function after a stroke by fooling the brain into thinking that the weak limb is working.

MRI - Magnetic Resonance Imaging

Multi Infarct Dementia (MID) - Long term confusion caused by a series of small strokes

Muscle Tone - Also known as *tonus* -the continuous and passive partial contraction of the muscles or the muscle's resistance to passive stretch during a resting state

- **Low tone is** experienced as "floppy, mushy, dead weight; and
- **High tone is** experienced as "light, tight, and strong "Muscles with **high tone** are not necessarily strong, and muscles with **low tone** are not necessarily weak.
- In general, **low tone** does increase flexibility and decrease strength and **high tone** does decrease flexibility and increase strength.

Muscle Tension - Muscles of the body remain semi-contracted for a period of time in the resting state.

Naso-gastric (NG) - A tube that is inserted through the nostril of a patient into the stomach to feed a Dysphagic patient

Neurologist - A physician specialising in neurology and trained to investigate or diagnose and treat neurological disorders

Neuroplasticity - Neuro *(brain)* Plasticity *(pliability)* is a term used to describe the changeability for the brain to relearn, even in adulthood

NMES - Neuromuscular Electrical Stimulation

Nystagmus - Involuntary jerking of the eyes

Occupational therapy - Is the use of assessment and treatment to develop, recover, or maintain the daily living and work skills of people with physical, mental, or cognitive disorders.

Partial Anterior Circulation Syndrome (PACS) -The medical classification of a stroke at the front of the brain which is caused by an infarct

Patent Foramen Ovale (PFO) - A hole in the heart that did not close the way it should have after birth

Paralysis - Loss of muscle function for one or more muscles

Permissive Hypertension - A strategy where blood pressure is allowed to rise for a short period of time to ensure that damaged brain tissues receive enough blood flow. Usually no more than 24 to 48 hours

Percutaneous Endoscopic Gastrostomy (PEG) - The insertion of a tube into the wall of the stomach to feed Dysphagic patients

Platelets - Colourless blood cells that help the blood to clot.

Pneumonia - An infection in one or both of the lungs.

Post Stroke Fatigue - Often confused with the

misconception of being tired and lazy.

Positive Emission Tomography(PET) -A detailed scan of the brain

Physiotherapy - Is a physical medicine and rehabilitation speciality that remediates impairments and promotes mobility, function, and quality of life through examination, diagnosis, prognosis, and physical intervention

Posterior Circulation Syndrome (POCS) -The medical classification of a stroke at the back of the brain which is caused by an infarct

Pseudobulbar Affect (PBA) - Emotional liability resulting in uncontainable outbursts of laughter or crying for no reason

Psychologist - A professional trained to evaluate behavioural and mental disorders

Pulmonary Embolism (PE) - A blockage of an artery in the lungs caused by blood clots that travel from elsewhere in the body.

Repetition - The act of repeating over and over

Rehabilitation - Specialised healthcare dedicated to improving, maintaining or restoring physical strength, cognition and mobility with maximised results[6]

Seizure - A sudden uncontrollable electrical disturbance in the brain

SCD (Sickle Cell Disease) - A red blood cell disorder where a sudden defective protein causes the red blood cells to become stiff and sticky instead of flexible and form a sickle (C shape) or a crescent.

Small vessel disease - The thickening and disease of tiny arteries deep in the brain reducing the flow of oxygen-rich blood

Stenosis - Narrowing of an artery due to plaque build-up within the artery.

Stroke - occurs when there is poor blood flow to the brain. There are two types of strokes:

- **Haemorrhagic stroke -** when a blood vessel in the brain ruptures
- **Ischaemic stroke-** where a blood vessel is blocked, restricting blood flow
- **Subarachnoid Haemorrhage** - A ruptured blood vessel that is bleeding into the space surrounding the brain

Spasticity - Is a feature of altered skeletal muscle performance with a combination of paralysis, increased tendon reflex activity and hypertonia; It is also commonly referred to as an unusual "tightness", stiffness, or "pull" of muscles.

Speech Therapy - Specialises in evaluating and treating communication disorders, voice disorders, and swallowing disorders.

Subluxation of the Shoulder - Partial or incomplete dislocation of the shoulder

TBI - Traumatic Brain Injury. A stroke is classified as a TBI

TENS - Transcutaneous Electrical Nerve Stimulation

Thalamus - The section of the brain that deals with sensation

Transient Ischemic Attack (TIA) - AKA a mini-stroke. Caused by a clot, they are transient (temporary), lasting less than 24 hours

Thrombolysis - A Clot-busting drug that is used to dissolve a blood clot which is causing an Ischaemic Stroke

Thrombosis - Blockage in a blood vessel due to a blood clot

Thrombus - A blood clot that forms in a vessel and remains there.

Total serum cholesterol - A combined measurement of a person's high-density lipoprotein (HDL) and low-density lipoprotein (LDL).

Total Anterior Circulation Syndrome (TACS) - The medical classification for a large stroke at the front of the brain caused by an Infarct

Vasospasm - occurs when a blood vessel narrows,

blocking blood flow

Vertebral arteries - A major artery on either side of the neck that runs through the spinal column in the neck and supplies blood to the back of the brain and spine.

Vertigo - Abnormal sensation of movement, dizziness

Brian Maram

About the Author

AUTHOR'S NAME: Brian Maram

Website: www.neuvare.com

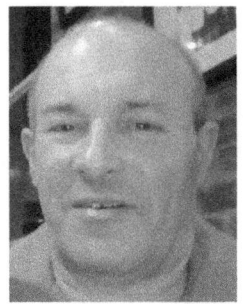 At the tender age of Eighteen, the author survived a head-on collision when a drunk driver failed to stop at an intersection and collided with him head-on.

The force of the impact caused the dashboard to be pushed further back into the car's cab, causing the steering wheel to collide with his face. He was instantly knocked unconscious. The force of the impact was so great that it bent the steering wheel and embedded it an inch into the dashboard.

Lucky to be alive, he was rushed to hospital and into an operating theatre where they strategically reassembled all the broken bones in his face. After the emergency operation, he was placed in ICU and into an induced coma. The impact had caused the author to suffer a Traumatic Brain Injury.

The following years were pure hell for his family, and after numerous operations, he made a full recovery.

Other Books By Brian Maram

- The stroke survivors Handbook
- Through The Eyes of a Survivor - Stroke

Can I Ask A Favour?

If you enjoyed this book, found it useful or otherwise then I'd appreciate it if you would post a short review on Amazon. I do read all the reviews personally so that I can continually write what people are wanting.

If you'd like to leave a review then please scan the QR Code below to visit the link:

Thanks for your support!

www.ingramcontent.com/pod-product-compliance
Lightning Source LLC
Chambersburg PA
CBHW072211170526
45158CB00002BA/540